Finding Balance in Today's Chaotic World

A Guide to Finding Ease and Stillness

Alana Kennedy

Introduction

I genuinely love seeing people happy. Stress-free, thriving, being loved, and having that glow on their faces. I love it when people are soft with themselves and do the kinds of things that make their hearts smile. I love it when people immerse themselves and dip their toes in puddles of delight; when they walk away from things that don't in any way wish them well. I love it when people are unapologetic about living lives on their own terms, paving a way for themselves even if it does not make sense for others out there; this kind of happiness looks good on everyone and it's the kind I certainly wish upon you.

A couple of years ago, my life took a completely unexpected U-turn. I got into a tragic bicycle accident and life, as I had known and experienced it, was no longer the same. Gone were the days when I could go cycling up in the mountains, filling my lungs with the fresh, untainted air from up there. I fell into a deep, dark, and bottomless pit during those months when I was in recovery from my back surgery. Why me? What did I do to deserve this? Surely, I must've been dreaming. I'd think to myself. It was just too painful a reality to accept.

Months later, things got slightly better. I found a job that allowed me to work remotely from home, but boy oh boy did I not know what was in store for me. Things were a mess. People say that you have more autonomy when you work from home. Surely, I must've been doing something wrong because that was not how I had come to experience it. There was always stuff lying all around, with my somber mood, my chronic pain, needing to make time for my family (who I love dearly), and my dog, I felt like I could explode! Things needed to change; I needed to change because if I didn't, I would disintegrate. Break up into a million pieces and never find myself whole again.

The day was a Tuesday, somewhere between 9 and 10:30 a.m., and I felt that I needed a change of scenery. There's this quirky old coffee shop that's roughly a 10-minute drive from my house. They play old folk music and have a kaleidoscope of sweet treats that awaken a childlike excitement within; the entire place and its atmosphere feel like a hug from a grandma. Warm, inviting, and smells like cinnamon and spice—I love it.

The whole idea was to go there and get a bit of work done. I was days behind deadlines, and I knew that if I still wanted to be employed by the end of that week, I'd have to get a move on. Fast-forward to a couple of minutes later, I still haven't gotten much done. Instead, I found myself people-watching. There was one lady who caught my eye. She looked unbothered. At that moment, the slow simplicity of being in a coffee shop, watching as people scurried back and forth between the places they needed to be, thinking about nothing and everything all at once seemed like enough; Like everything in this lifetime was just pure... magic.

There are way too many of us who do not know how to be still and savor a moment. Too many of us are getting suffocated by our own chaos. You could be at the dinner table with your family but have a series of thoughts swimming through your mind. Did you pay for the kid's aftercare or piano lessons? Are you going to have enough time to stop by the dry cleaners tomorrow after work? What are you going to cook tomorrow for dinner after work? Or wear it to the corporate dinner tomorrow evening? What about the present moment... The ones where you get to listen to your partner tell you all about their day? Does your little one tell you about the frogs that they caught today at playtime? The moments where you engage in meaningless banter about which ice cream flavor is best, or which basketball team is winning the game over the next coming weekend. Don't you think that these moments matter more than crossing another item off your to-do list?

There seem to be never-ending demands for our time. There's always an extra email that needs to be responded to. One more report needs to be mailed. Another appointment. Another commitment. It just won't stop. There's always time for them, but what about you? Where do you fit in? Where is that space for you? Most importantly, what do you want to create space for amongst all of this?

A life of balance is a life that takes all the elements of your life, pieces them together, and like a mosaic, brings to life a work of art that is understood by you alone. A balanced life is a collection of experiences, lessons, failures, and successes that help you get to know who you are; it's when everything comes together, and you realize that you don't have to have to be everything all at once to everyone. That you are allowed to say no and not feel guilty about it.

Together, we're going to navigate and figure out what a balanced life looks like to you. It's fun. It's full of surprises. Some are pleasant and some, not so much. It's a process that is really going to pull you outside of your comfort zone and stretch you (emotionally, mentally, and physically) in the best ways possible. There are questions that you'll be asked, questions that might challenge the reality that you are living in right now; questions that won't even make sense until you put them into practice.

You are here right now, and that means that something spectacular is waiting for you just around the bend. The distant things that you've always wanted to prioritize are going to become just that... priorities. You are finally going to figure out who you are, and that'll help you become the better mom, dad, sister, or brother that you've always wanted to become. It'll definitely feel as if the whole universe is conspiring in your favor—that is what intention does after all. It gathers up all that is meant to be yours and lines it perfectly in your way.

I'm honored that you chose me as your partner in change. The one who gets to see you gets to help you find those remarkable things about your life—a life that you can enjoy and that you are fully satisfied with. Take a highlighter, your sticky notes, and a couple of extra pens while you are at it. We're about to open up Pandora's box of discoveries. You owe it to yourself, and all that you have been, to discover what is ready to spill out for you.

Chapter 1: It Starts Right Here

So much of our lives revolve around walking around and drawing up lists of things that need to be done, things to patch up, and holes to fill. How about as of right now, you start walking through your life to uncover its full potential?

My mother, a very wise woman indeed, once told me I should do things for myself—even when I don't feel like it. Climbing out of your comfort zone or choosing to go against the status quo will require a whole lot of willpower and a change in mindset. We have to be willing to let go of the idea that things have to be a certain way, or that they should be perfectly aligned. Every step that we take to expand our comfort zones is a step closer to personal growth, lifelong learning, and fulfillment.

To find ourselves, we're going to have to start thinking for ourselves... Knowing where you are currently positioned in your life and where you want to go, seems like the best possible place to start when doing your life audit, surprisingly enough, however, that is a question that far too many of us battle to answer. That's why a life audit is necessary for these instances. A life audit is a comprehensive assessment of your life that helps you determine what actions you need to take based on the situation you are facing. It's a process that requires vulnerability from you. It's a beautiful process but can also be devilishly messy as well. It's about being transparent and not leaving any stone unturned. It's about deepening our understanding of ourselves and our lives. It's a challenging thing to be honest with yourself about where you are because the answers that come up are ones that don't always match up with what we want.

So how and where exactly do you begin when starting your life audit?

You start by rounding up all the areas in your life where you want to make all those necessary changes. So, you set time aside and inspect all of those areas that take up your time, your money, and your mental, emotional, and physical energy. There's probably way too much on your plate—which makes it easy for the disconnect to go unnoticed. Finding those areas where the disconnect begins can equip you with the knowledge that you need to start managing your expectations, how you can start enforcing boundaries and setting goals that matter to you and where you want to be in life. Some of the areas that you can focus your attention on include:

- **Your lifestyle in general:**

  o Am I content with the life that I have and am living right now?

  o What makes me feel fulfilled and alive?

  o What achievements am I most proud of?

  o Where are most of my time and energy invested?

- **Your physical health**

  o Have you been eating healthy and nourishing your body with wholesome and enriching kinds of foods?

  o Have you been meeting your daily water intake goals?

  o Have you at least gone on a walk or moved in a way that helps you relieve the tension caused by daily life stressors?

  o Am I getting enough daily rest and finding healthy ways to destress?

  o How does my body feel after having my meals, do I feel bloated, lethargic, or energized?

- **Mental health**

  o How have I been feeling lately? Have I been engaged or a little distant from everyone and everything around me?

○ Where have my stress levels been lately?

○ Is there anything that I need to talk about or need to get off my chest?

○ What can I do for myself to feel a little bit better?

○ Is there anything that I have been worried about lately?

○ Have I been doing enough and investing in things that bring me a sense of joy?

○ When was the last time I paid myself a compliment and appreciated tiny little things about myself?

○ When was the last time I laughed—genuinely laughed until my tummy started to hurt?

● **Family and relationships**

○ Have I been investing some time in nurturing the relationships with my closest ones?

○ When was the last time I had an open and honest conversation with a friend, a sibling, or a partner?

○ In what ways can I provide support to those who I love and those who love me?

○ Am I happy with the quality of my emotional and intellectual intimacy with my connections?

○ Do the people around me make me feel supported and seen?

○ Are they the giver or the taker?

○ Am I the giver or the taker?

○ How are these people making me feel about myself? Do our interactions leave me feeling drained or energized?

- **Career and finance**

○ Am I happy with the career that I currently have?

○ Do I have a healthy emergency fund savings account?

○ Do I spend money recklessly and make a lot of impulsive purchases?

○ Do I know where my money is going at the end of each month?

○ When was the last time I inspected my bank statements? Are there unnecessary subscriptions and expenses that I should consider letting go of?

○ Do I have a retirement fund so that I can make regular contributions?

Reflection is productive. The deepest and most significant changes begin with self-reflection; it's about choosing to react differently to the same old behaviors we used to exhibit. One thing that I believe is that the universe will always be asking us if we're ready to stop engaging with old habits so that we can enter that parallel life that we've always been looking for. Reflection is the only way that you are going to learn to really get to know yourself. Consider this for a moment: Hiring managers ask candidates a series of questions to get to know who they are before presenting an offer. The same rule applies to personal reflection as well.

We won't get to that divine destination if we do not know where we stand with ourselves.

Once you've had that conversation with yourself, the one that prompts you to shift the narrative of how you've always seen things, you start building, and the best place to start is by uncovering your values.

Uncovering Your Values

Knowing what your values are will help you live on purpose; even through life's most trying seasons. The right set of values is the one that is best aligned with your vision of a beautiful life. They're what help us create an authentic life that works in conjunction, instead of against our wiring. They're what allow us to be unapologetically alive, unafraid to let our lights shine bright, and journey through life with wholeness and joy.

If I walked up to you at this moment and asked you what it is that you value, what would you say? Would you take a moment to pause and then moments later begin replaying them to me as if they were the lyrics to your favorite song, or would it look a little like a game of touch and go? Are you grappling to find a definite answer that fits perfectly in your palms?

It's overwhelming to start from scratch, especially if you are not all that certain where to begin, or how to even begin. But rest assured, as with all other things in life, once you move a few feet beyond that starting point, it becomes a whole lot easier. Let's go all out to find that starting point.

Naming your value words

The best place to start when looking to define your valuable words is to look for the roots of what is most important to you. What is it that sets your soul alight? What elements of your life make you wake up and immediately think: *Oh, yes! I'm so glad to have made it to another day. I am so grateful to be able to experience this moment, this life as me.*

If you can't yet find the answer to that, think about what it is that you *do not* want. I personally find it a lot easier to weed out the things that I know do not belong, and then from there, I carefully start rearranging things in a way that feels aligned.

Find those three to four words that really resonate with you; the words that you would feel most proud to guide your decisions.

Here is a list of value words that you can use to get yourself started:
- honesty
- simplicity
- compassion
- humility
- intuition
- gratitude
- meaningfulness
- progress
- independence
- balance
- bravery
- Confidence
- respect
- integrity
- authenticity
- balance

Looking at this list, it might occur to you that all of these names are of significance to you. It's okay, in that situation, I want you to look for the ones that are always on the forefront of your mind which will give you an indication of what values you hold near and dearest to your heart.

Look for them in the people who you admire the most

We tend to see ourselves or the person that we want to be reflected in the people who we admire. Create another list with the names of your role models or people who inspire you. You could start off with a classmate, a colleague whose passion and spirit you admire. Or a well-known figure. What is it about them that draws you to them? Is it their authenticity, their quirks, honesty, or the way they treat people?

Look at how far you've come

Pain, heartache, victories, and disappointment are our greatest teachers. Think about those moments of your life that you didn't think you were capable of surviving or the moments that made you feel like you were floating on clouds; moments where blessings in abundance came gushing right your way. What were your reactions? How did you treat those around you? Perhaps in that moment of victory, you might have come to realize that humility is more important, or modesty matters to you when put in the spotlight. And in those instances of misfortune, you might have learned that kindness matters most to you, and in times of struggle, you never want anyone to feel as if they're alone and have to carry their burdens all on their own.

Connect them to key areas in your personal life

Your values are that map that helps you navigate relationships, friendships, work, and your mental and physical health. So, when you take a look into those different areas. Are they a reflection of your life's personal mission statement? Do they honor that promise that you made to yourself? As someone who values simplicity and doesn't like for my life to be unnecessarily uncomplicated for myself, it's been pretty helpful to have something to go back to as a reference check to help me simplify more.

Put them into practice

Words are much easier to take in when written on a sheet of paper, aren't they? Holding ourselves accountable, following up, and checking in to see whether we're actively applying these values to our lives in everyday situations is the hard part. Let's say you are part of a group of friends who always want to be in on every latest trend. What do you do when they ask you when you are changing the model of your car, or when you are getting the latest version of a phone? Do head on up to the store to take part in their endless game of "Keeping up on the Jones," or do you assert yourself by letting them know that you are content with the simplicity of your life as it is?

Re-visit and reevaluate

My favorite part of getting to this life thing is that I am constantly changing. I am not who I was six months ago, and three months from now, I certainly won't be the same person either. When you change, things that mattered to you a couple of months ago will not necessarily matter as much to you now. Change is a divine thing and we should always be waiting to welcome it with open arms. There may be that occasional moment of worry about what lies on the other side of it, but believe me, I like to believe it's all things good.

Chapter 2: Decluttering Your Life

It's easy to think that clutter is just clutter. But the actual truth is that our clutter is often a symptom of something else that we'd rather not face. The clutter surrounding your physical space may be a sign that you are lonely and still need to find yourself. Emotional clutter that you are holding on to may be a sign that there are issues within and around you that need to be dealt with. Time clutter, your packed schedule, your endless march of to-do, and things that you just cannot miss, might be a sign of the loneliness that you are living with.

Clutter... There's a heaviness that clings to the words. Something that suggests isolation, loneliness, and perhaps even frustration?

We tend to assume that filling our lives with "more" will bring us more joy, contentment, and satisfaction. But The truth is that clutter only prevents us from being the best we can be. More of everything means less of you for you.

Clutter manifests itself in different ways. It's in the space around us. The closets are overflowing with multiple items of clothing. Shelves that are lined with knick-knacks that hold no significance or don't mean all that much. It's in our garages that no longer hold space for our cars, but items that were accumulated over the years out of fear of being left behind.

It's in our electronic devices. Thousands of unread emails flood our inboxes. The apps take up storage space but are hardly ever used.

It can be found in our fears that we carry around with us like dead weight waiting to be shed. The limiting beliefs that hold you back. "I can't do that"; "I'm not smart enough"; "I'm not talented enough." It's a lack of peace of mind. Holding on too tightly to the past.

Clutter Isn't always easy to spot. It isn't always loud, but you'll know it's there. You'll feel it in the way that discomfort pulls at the strings of your heart.

The real goal should be to have just enough for you to be able to see the value that the things add. Just enough without having to give up your time, or extra space. Just Enough so that you have more time and energy to invest in living and being alive.

What Clutter Is Doing to You

It's robbing you of precious time and moments. Everything you own also owns a portion of your time because you have to—at some point—set time aside to work for the money to buy it, to care for it, and to keep it in good condition. It all seems inconsequential when it's out like this, but those fifteen, ten, and twenty minutes add up after a while, and that's why it sometimes feels as though you can't catch a break.

The limiting beliefs that you have as well are preventing you from building meaningful relationships for yourself. Imagine all that you'd achieve if you started giving more yeses to courage instead of fear. Imagine where you'd be and how much prouder you'd be of yourself.

It creeps into your relationships. When all of your time goes to work, trying to manage *things* the people you love are naturally going to be on the shorter end when it comes to receiving love and affection. That comes from having to keep these *things*—resentment, anger, and frustration toward the ones you love. That's what causes people to drift away from one another. You won't ever be able to dedicate your whole self if parts of you are owned by meaningless possessions.

Clutter interferes with how much pleasure you get to derive from life. If your lines aren't clearly defined, then nothing will ever feel like enough. Contentment comes from being at ease, and at peace with where you are and what you have right now. If that is something that you have to be okay with. I'm not saying that this means that you shouldn't want to move forward or progress in life. I'm just saying that it shouldn't take away from the beauty of being here *right now.*

It keeps us imprisoned in our own lives. Freedom is an exhale. It's looking all around you and not feeling stifled. It's the gift of not feeling like you are boxed or having to be anything other than who you already are. It's kicking off your shoes and running barefoot and wildly into the great big unknown. It's saying to yourself. I'm scared and not all that certain about what lies ahead, but I'm going to run toward it either way.

When we hold on to clutter, we latch on to expectations and identities of ourselves that we think we should be. In some way, we're telling ourselves that it's not okay to change or embrace the glorious now. Clutter is heavy, and when things are heavy, they slow us down and stunt the progress that we are capable of making. When you feel like you are never catching up or making any progress, you are going to remain stuck in negative thinking patterns that prevent you from seeing the possibilities of what is.

To unpack and lessen the load that clutter has, you have to understand what it does to you and what it certainly doesn't. Clutter steals from us, and I believe that in itself should be motivation for us to protect ourselves, and our emotional, physical, and spiritual valuables from finding ourselves in the hands of the enemy.

Take a moment and consider how the different types of clutter affect you in life, love, and your career. Which one do you feel most compelled to rid yourself of? Where would you like to see yourself move from that point onward? The great news for you is that we'll be looking into how we can do complete resets; together, we're going to run toward clarity, away from all the noise and excess.

Unpacking Our Emotional Clutter

What is inside emotional clutter and what about it makes it so particularly dangerous?

The physical clutter, the one that's easiest to spot with our bare eyes, is also the one that's easiest to deal with. The one that lies beneath the surface; the one that creeps up on you on a Sunday Morning and shows up as uncontrollable sobs, or a panic attack in the middle of your kitchen, is one that is terrifying to look in the eyes. It's years of pent-up rage that boils over unexpectedly all so suddenly. It's the anxiety that stops you in your tracks at the grocery store and makes you forget what you came there to buy. It's fear that shows up in a moment of euphoria and whispers darkly to you: *What if, moments from now, all of this is taken away from you?*

What makes it particularly difficult to address is that as a society, we've never really asked each other: "How are you," and waited long enough to hear the unembellished answer. The answer is beyond "I'm fine" or "I've never been better." I guess the "I'm struggling right now" or "I'm holding on, but I will slip soon enough," are too honest. Too close to the heart; they're the answers that cross the lines of what's comfortable.

It's okay to feel anything that is less than okay. Perfection is overrated and what is it in any way? Those less-than–okay-feelings are a normal part of life. We shouldn't deny their existence; it's the denial that makes them defy us and catch us off guard when we least expect it (and not in a good way).

The most common types of emotional clutter are:

- **Anxiety and fear**

You've conceptualized a beyond-brilliant idea. It's something that you've been working on for months – perhaps even years – something that you know will transform lives far beyond your own, but when the time comes to start putting action where your words are, that voice comes in, the voice that tells you that you don't and will never measure up. The voice that asks you how dare you have the audacity to be? Anxiety and fear are incapacitated. When we don't work through them and ask ourselves *why* they're there and where they come from. We subject ourselves to a lifetime of slavery toward them. I knew a long time ago that I wanted to write this book for you. Sure, I had those moments when I thought to myself that there are billions of other talented writers, so who would want to read anything that I wrote? But in that same moment, it dawned on me that those other writers aren't me – that's where the difference is. Is it easy to write a book? *No.* Is it always an enjoyable experience? Not quite because it's a creative process that stretches and tests you and your limits and I love that.

Your dreams and desires deserve to be given an identity of their own. They deserve every ounce of the spotlight. That's why it's important to shovel through those fears. To befriend the discomfort and let you guide you to a better place.

● Guilt

The *could haves* and the *should haves* are something else, aren't they? Remembering our misses and misfortunes makes us slip into dark emotional places. Places where a series of negative self-talk stems; a place that does nothing but drags you and makes you feel unworthy. Obsessing over past circumstances that you have no power of caning is unhelpful. You can't tie your identity or your worth to moments and places that have long come and gone. Another way guilt makes an appearance in our lives is through our over-commitments. You missed someone's housewarming party because of something that was way beyond your control and now you feel compelled to go to that Friday night barbeque that they invited you to, even though you know that you'll be drained – physically and emotionally—after a long day of work.

So, you go forth with the yes that you actually want to be a no because we have to be there for people, isn't it?

● Anger

This is a tough one. How do you let it slide when someone wrongs or hurts you in the worst ways imaginable? How do we move away from that trauma? It really is a lot easier to be angry, but what we don't realize is that the anger ends up doing a lot more damage to us than the person who we're holding it against. It hurts us more because it clouds our judgment; we end up holding it against the innocent soul. It prevents you from moving forward and building more meaningful connections. Letting go of anger shouldn't be about whether the person that you are holding it against deserves it or not. It should be about you; about getting yourself to an emotionally healthy place so that you can be healthier and happier.

- **Denial**

Some things are difficult to accept as they are and validly so. It is a coping mechanism for most of us. Sometimes it helps to blindly believe that something isn't a problem – until it explodes and creates an even bigger problem. If you choose to go through life without acknowledging the tough things. You are not going to feel any happier. You are going to feel powerless in your own life. Owning our struggles and choosing to be active participants to change, regardless of how difficult it is, is how we take that power back. How we reclaim control and put ourselves back in the driver's seat.

Tips For Dealing With Emotional Clutter

Think about a hiking trail. Doesn't it become a lot easier to navigate the path the more times you walk it? The uphill becomes less daunting for you. The bushes, the scenery around, dirt, and rocks along the path become less foreign and a lot more like friends who are there to help you navigate the unfamiliar. This is how our minds operate as well. The more we explore, the more fearless we become, and the easier it becomes to step into distant places. You have the power to change your perspective of how you think about the negatives.

Tip 1: Familiarize yourself with the kind of clutter that you are dealing with

Your ability to identify the type of clutter can be the making or breaking point of your journey. You have to be able to separate the trash from the treasure and distinguish between the momentary feelings (i.e., anxiety about test results that you are awaiting, and the more complex emotional layers. The fears of abandonment, the never-ending cycles of negative self-talk. You can use the pointers that we made above about the different types of clutter.

Tip 2: Don't be afraid to ask for help

Some battles aren't ours to fight on our own... That's why it's okay to ask for help from a professional or someone who knows better. There are certain aspects of healing such as getting closure or moving on, that require us to get a perspective from someone else who can help us see the situation differently. Life through our own lens is sometimes only black or white, but gray matters too. We need it to help us understand how we are sometimes the greatest contributors to our own pain.

Tip 3: Do a little bit of work every day

The overwhelm that comes from a lifetime of unresolved/ unaddressed emotion, is not going to be resolved in a day, or a week. It takes months and some time in certain situations, years too. So, make the commitment to connect to your psyche daily. If anger is the one emotion that is holding you back and preventing you from living a life that is rooted in joy, why not try committing to doing at least one thing that brings you joy on a daily basis? These little acts that bring more joy and contentment into your life will bring more satisfaction into your life. If fear is something that you are struggling with, practice bringing in the smallest acts of courage into your day—little things like going out for a walk all on your own. Say hello to a stranger. Practice asking for help in your most vulnerable situations. It really is the smallest things that make all the difference.

Tip 4: Make time for emotional and mental rest

Rest is not wasted potential or time thrown away. Have some hot tea or coffee and walk underneath an overcast sky. Go pick some flowers in your garden. Bake a cake, have a slice, or two, and eat them as if that is the last thing that you will ever get to do in this lifetime. Find a moment and press yourself in those seconds. Moments of purpose and pleasure are what make our emotional clutter a lot easier to deal with.

Tip 5: Mind the media that you consume

The things that we see passed all across the internet can be easily mistaken as "normal". This so-called state of being connected is exactly what is distancing us from our values. Time away from social media platforms is exactly what we need to help us reconnect with our identity. Turn down the digital noise and let your soul find its way back to the native home that belongs to it in your heart.

Tip 6: Be more decisive

When faced with too many options, we tend to procrastinate because of a phenomenon called decision fatigue. The best way to combat this is to start giving yourself a time limit when faced with decisions to make. This way you'll avoid putting things off and letting your anxiety over the choices that you have spilled over to the following day.

When it comes to matters of the mind, it's important to engrave the idea within us that we do not have to believe everything that our mind tells us is true. So, practice. Practice telling yourself that you are going to be okay, and soon enough the "I can't handle this on my own," will turn into "I have made it to shore; even when I thought I was drowning and felt that the waves would carry me with them. So, I know that this too is not permanent."

The Physical Clutter

Stuff, glorious stuff... What category would you say you fall under when you look at the space around you: the one who's got too many unnecessary, just enough, or not enough? These categories are rather subjective because "enough" is relative. But I'm going to take a wild guess and assume that because you are here, reading this book, you likely fall under the category of the individual who has "stuff" spilling out of their ears.

Letting go of physical clutter isn't as easy as chucking things in garbage bags and throwing them in the trash. For one, our stuff has sentimental value. So, letting them go means that we'll have to address the grief that comes from having held on to these things for too long. So, if you've been wondering where to start and how to even, I've got just the tips for you:

- You do it bit by bit. If you are new to decluttering, it's not exactly something that you are going to master in a day, so starting small and dedicating just as little as 10 to fifteen minutes a day, is how you build your momentum.

- Ask yourself some critical questions. Questions will help you figure out what clutter is and isn't to you. They're there to guide your practice and provide some direction to you.

  ○ Do you really love this item? "Good enough" is not a solid enough answer to keep holding on to something.

  ○ How frequently do I use this item? It's easy to assume that something is a necessity for you, but have you used it in the past 5 to 8 months? If the answer is no, then you don't really need it as much as you think you do. Just because something is useful, doesn't mean that you need it.

○ Do I want this item to be a part of my journey going forward? Decluttering is about sacrifice. You have to be willing to let certain things go so that there is sufficient room for the things that really do matter. You have a vision of how you want your life to look. Is this item one of the pieces of the puzzle that fits?

○ Are there similar items that perhaps serve the same purpose? I've noticed that most of the items that I own serve more than one purpose. You don't need one thousand different items.

○ Wouldn't it be better if I borrowed this item when I needed it? This question is especially helpful when it comes to bulky items that you only ever use once in a while. Say for instance you have a bread maker, and you only ever use it around Thanksgiving or Christmas time. Do you think it's a significant enough item to take up space in your house? Do you not have a friend or a daily who you can borrow it from when it is needed?

○ Is this something that I would buy again? If you were to ever lose or have the item break, would you consider buying it again? If the answer is yes, then it likely is something that is of value to you. If it's a no, then maybe you should consider letting it go.

○ Is there a place for it here or in other words, does it fit the vision of the lifestyle that you are creating right now? So, I mentioned that over time, all of us change and so do our likes and our dislikes, so some things are just not practical to keep with you anymore.

○ Does it hold any sentimental value? I think some people would hand me if they were to hear me say this, but sometimes we simply do not like the things that people give to us, in those situations, I think that it is okay to let the items go. It's the heart and mind where our memories are held, not in possessions or things.

○ Does it still work? A lot of us have a habit of keeping things with old holes or things that are no longer functioning. Faulty things end up taking up a lot of unnecessary space. So, word of advice, discard those old electrical appliances.

○ Did I even remember that I owned this item? It happens to the best of us, you open your cupboard, and out springs something you didn't know you had. If this happened to you, the chances are, you do not need this (this rule does not only apply to clothes.

○ If I suddenly had to uproot my life, would I take this item with me? Here's the thing: you can't take everything with you when you move. This approach helps you put into perspective what you can or cannot live without. If the item is something that you would not take with you, then you do not need it.

• Have an ongoing donation box. There will always be stuff you don't need that we'll always be useful to someone else. You can start off by asking some of your family members and if what you have to offer doesn't appeal to their tastes, take them to charity.

• Make time a non-negotiable date in your schedule. If decluttering is not something that you particularly enjoy, treat it as you would a date with an important client or a sibling that you wouldn't want to miss. You have to be able to hold yourself accountable if it is something that you are serious about doing.

- Have space boundaries. Decide how much space you want each of your items to take up. This will make it easier for you to prioritize what it is that you do and do not want to keep.

- Incorporate activities that bring you enjoyment during the process to make it feel less like a burden. For example, if dancing is something that you truly enjoy doing. Incorporate some music in the background. Or you could play a soothing podcast in the background. Decluttering should remind us that even the tough stuff can be fun.

- Keep track of what you are also bringing in as well. Life is cyclical. So, you are going to also have to guard yourself and be mindful of what you are also bringing back into your life. If you do limit your acquisition of things, you are going to find yourself in a never-ending cycle of decluttering. Something that you can do to limit the amount of stuff that you are bringing in includes:

  - Shopping bans. Committing to periods where you choose not to buy any new clothes or luxury accessories.

  - "One in, one out" rule. So, in essence, this just means that if you buy one thing, you have to get rid of something else.

I like to believe that "enough" rests somewhere in between having too much and just enough. There is always going to be a favorite item, something new that you just cannot live without, that is why it is self-love in the most radical of ways to look around you and make the conscious decision to not have it all. To deny yourself, to step back and realize that simpler is easier, better, and wiser.

The Digital Clutter

If you don't disconnect from your phone, you are going to disconnect from the world around you.

Before the age when cell phones were so popular, you could leave the workplace and actually leave work and not have to worry about new emails coming in at an unreasonable hour and having to instantly respond to them. You could actually leave work and leave it there where it is supposed to stay.

There is a freedom that cannot be explained when you give yourself the opportunity to switch off and retreat into a world of your own. Don't you think that giving yourself uninterrupted "me-time" to enjoy time with your family, to have time out in the sun or at the beach? You owe yourself that much, don't you think?

Switching Off

It can be awfully tempting to reach out for your phone every time the pang of notification goes off, or when the red light starts flashing, but true peace and contentment can be found in those moments when you ease yourself from the pressure of constantly having to be accessible and reachable to everyone around you.

It's important that we set boundaries with ourselves with our technological devices. Some things that you can do to create a little bit of distance between you and your technological devices include:

- **Setting curfews with yourself for cellphone use**. For example, you can establish a rule whereby you don't respond to texts or emails after a certain time in the evening.
- **Zone out certain areas of your house**. There are certain rooms where cell phones don't belong. Like the dining room for instance, when dining with your family, you shouldn't be too focused on what is happening in your virtual world.

Chapter 3: The Simple Art of Gratitude Finding

The change that beats within me recognizes the change happening all around me.

My work here on earth is to love all that exists around me without question or hesitation—the bees who are equal seekers of sweetness. The calm that exists in the waves of the ocean. The spicy flavors waft from my neighbor's kitchen as they prepare a hearty dinner for their family. My curious, awkward, and clumsy fingers. The eyes stand still and marvel at their surroundings in astonishment. The trees that rejoice, and the lips that sing of joy. This is gratitude and what it should feel like.

Gratitude—the magic word. I believe in it as much as I believe in the air that keeps us alive.

If you are looking for that immersive life experience, gratitude is certainly the way to go about life. It gives us perspective, it's a little scary sometimes because it can have us examining our deepest fears, our secrets, in a way that makes it feel devilishly good or us to be alive, all of that is possible because it makes us brave enough to open our hearts p a little wider than we ever would have considered. Is that not something to marvel at and be in awe of?

It is much easier to practice when things are going well for us. When things are aligning divinely in our favor. That is why it requires intentionality and practice, so that even through the rough patches. Having a mindset that is rooted in gratitude does not mean being ignorant of all the other things going on that you do not like. It's not ignoring your sadness, anxiety, your fear, or anger. It doesn't have to be a constant at every waking minute of your life. It won't be the same today as it is tomorrow. Being grateful does not mean that you have no capacity to feel anything else that does not have a close relationship to joy.

I believe that even when it's hard, we should all try to practice it every day because it gives us mindset shifts that we didn't know we needed. It gives you eyes to see the little, good things and not the bad that try to rob us of all our joy. When you start, it may seem like there's not much that's happening, but believe me, there is, over time, you'll start to see all that you'd taken for granted with much more clarity.

- **Not every day is going to be your favorite**. Some days will be heavy on the heart; some days will have you questioning if the strength that it took you to get to where you are right now is a phony one, but gratitude brings acceptance in as a contributing factor, and you start to realize that not every day is about being grateful, but about the power of choice—choosing to acknowledge that life gets a lot easier when you find at least one thing that is a blessing in your life.

- **Keep your focus on right now**. Here is a wonderful place to be. Practicing gratitude is what you need to keep you focused on the "right now." To make the most of what we have, these very moments that are sprinkled with joy, we have to keep our eyes focused on them. I am a futuristic person, always thinking about what potential tomorrow holds. My mind is constantly running at a thousand miles per hour, but when I remind myself that here is what matters, life starts to bloom beautifully right before my eyes.

Finding Ways to be Grateful Every Day

I wish for us the kinds of lives where we share stories with our families at three a.m. about the things that we used to do when we were younger. Stories about prioritizing life and all of those things that matter most to us without any hesitation. There are so many things in life, things that we take for granted, and most times, we don't even care to give those things a second glance. Like this moment right now, I am holed up in my cozy writing nook, wearing fuzzy socks, and indulging in a hot cup of cocoa. I am in my safe place. I am loved, well-taken care of, and living a life that someone I may not know wishes he had. I can spend my mornings laughing, loving, and being loved. I wouldn't know such bliss if I didn't make gratitude an everyday part of my life.

● **Gratitude journal.** Imagine what it would do for your life if you woke up every day and gave thanks for the little things, the big things, and everything else that falls in between. The more you fill your life with things you can find to be grateful for, the happier you'll be. When you sit down each morning and write about the people, the things, and events that you can be grateful for, you'll realize that on most occasions, the best things in life are those that are completely free.

Gratitude journal prompts

○ Write about people who you are particularly grateful to have in your life.

○ Write about something that made you laugh until your stomach hurt, or until you had tears in your eyes.

○ An important life lesson you've learned and what about it has been so significant to your being and making it to the place you are now.

○ A memory that transports you back to some of the greatest parts of your life.

○ A gift that you've received that you'll never forget.

○ A book that you've loved reading.

○ Your favorite time of day and why it's so special to you.

○ The people who you consider to be your family.

○ Something that you find magical about the universe.

○ Food you enjoy or conjures up memories that leave you feeling all warm and fuzzy on the inside.

○ Someone's gesture that made your day.

○ Modern conveniences that make your life much easier.

○ Talents that make you unique and separate you from the crowd.

○ Something different today, that wasn't all that good a year ago.

● **Create a "thank you" jar.** Three years ago, on New Year's Eve, I found an empty jar, and I promised myself that whenever something cool, hilarious, or unexpected happened to me, I'd write it down on a piece of paper, and close it off by saying thank you and slip it into the jar. The practice evolved over the years because I realized that some days, from their perspective, were pretty mundane and uneventful, so I'd write: "Today, I made it to the end of the day. Thank you, God, for carrying me to see the end of it."

When you feel your energy shifting throughout the day from high to low, you can reach out to the jar as a source of comfort. You'll remember the sweet old lady who slipped a tulip in your hand. The fun night out that you had with your friends catching up over cheap wine and laughing about blind dates that went wrong. These are the things that often seem trivial, and insignificant, so when things go wrong, you'll have endless reminders of how wonderful life can be when you intentionally chase after joy, day in and day out.

● **Give**. Generosity is a lifestyle. Nothing beats the sheer goodness of giving without expecting anything back in return. Also, giving isn't only just about us, it's also about the person that's receiving – it's about reminding them that there is still some goodness in the world. It's about reminding them that they do not have to do life alone. That we are here for them, and that as long as we have people to support us—even if they aren't family—we'll be alright.

Ways to Give

- **Time**: time is something that we all have, and we all can give some of it. This could be like offering to babysit your friends' children so that they can enjoy their date night together. Cooking a meal for a friend who's been way too busy. Volunteering at a local children's home, animal shelter, or sports club.

- **Your talents**: Our talents are not just for us, but for the world around us. There's something that you have within you that could help someone else. If you are a gifted speaker or an encourager, why not use that to reach out to someone and offer an uplifting word – words are medicine for a broken spirit. You never know what internal wars someone is fighting to survive, that word of motivation may just be what they need to convince their spirit to stay and fight it out to see another day.

- **Touch**: Reaching out doesn't usually cost us anything: being kind to the cashier packaging your groceries. Sending a thoughtful message to a friend or a colleague, leaving a sticky note reminder on a colleague's desk to remind them of their purpose. Kindness doesn't require extravagance, only genuine gestures that leave people with something meaningful, even if it cannot be seen with their eyes. If it can be felt with the heart, it's significant enough.

- **Treasures**: You can be generous with what you have been gifted. Take time, look at your finances or things that you have that you no longer use, and ask: how can I be a good steward of these blessings? Pay it forward and pay for someone's coffee during your morning coffee run. Donate some of your old clothes, sponsor someone, or buy groceries for someone who is less fortunate than you are. Generosity will not fail to draw light and abundance in your direction, it'll help you find yourself and people who are on the same path that you are on.

- **Practice presence**: You can be here, but not really be here. Presence is what allows us to experience the fullness of being alive.

Presence is love, we all deserve love, don't you think? It's so easy to overlook the beauty of presence in our fast-paced, technologically-driven lives, when that happens we miss out on the divine opportunity to receive the moments of our lives as is, but when you gather and cultivate that connection with the moment right now, to wholeheartedly appreciate life as it is, you strengthen and regenerate the field of goodness that is around you.

Ways to be More Present

- **Use your phone less**: In essence, spend a little less time on social media, and more time doing the things that you love; more rewarding activities... Things that won't have you comparing yourself to anyone else.

- **Connect with your surroundings**: So, instead of checking our phones every minute, we can go outside and notice how the clouds change shape. See Mother Nature for who she is and what she does. Notice her and allow her to help you witness the energy flow within you. An energy that leads to a profound clarity.

- **Be an active participant in the lives of those that you care about**: Be there when you are with your people. Listen to them, and all the silly things that they have to say. Be intentional with your eye contact, don't interrupt them when they are saying something, and let them finish speaking. They'll feel appreciated, and validated, and you'll feel much better about yourself as well.

- **Stop trying to multitask**: I get it. You may think that you are a superhuman and that you can do a million things all at once, but here's the thing, you won't hinge properly if your attention is divided between a lot of things. Focus on one thing and do that one thing well. What is in a label? Not juggling more than one thing at once does not make you any less of a significant being.

- **Take your beaks**: It doesn't make you lazy or any less dedicated to what you are doing. On the contrary, it is what can help make you ten times better. When you rest, you are essentially dodging all of the stress, burnout, and fatigue that comes from overworking yourself. Put a reminder on your phone if you have to. Work can wait for your wellness, can't.

You Can Be Grateful

Look around you and you will find that there is no shortage of blessings all around you. You don't have to wait for something to be taken away from you for you to recognize the value that it has in your life. Maybe you are going through the most today and can't seem to find those rays of light. If that is what you are feeling right now, here is a list of simple gratitude reminders to keep you anchored:

○ The fact that you made it through yesterday to see today.

○ You are holding this book in your hands; a book that is created to remind you to keep fighting for your life.

○ The people in life who taught you who you do not want to be around.

○ Meaningful compliments and conversations that make your cup an overflow of good.

○ The people who encourage you to keep going.

○ A peaceful morning where you get to celebrate and enjoy being alive.

○ The memories that hold a special place in your heart.

○ The inspiration that comes when you allow your mind to roam and wander freely.

○ Music that makes you want to dance.

○ Long, peaceful walks in nature.

○ Moments in time when everything flows and aligns perfectly as it should.

○ The air you breathe.

○ Your health.

○ Having a body that you are able to move.

○ Mother Nature.

○ Having a place that you can call your home.

○ Everything in between that makes you uniquely you.

Gratitude will always meet you where you are. It doesn't really matter how far you think you are, that is what makes it so particularly beautiful. Don't stop searching.

Chapter 4: Perfect Stillness

As much as we embrace the creative pursuits in our lives, may we equally embrace our soul-care activities: sitting, being still, pondering, and restoring our souls.

Stillness is about refreshing the body, the mind, and the soul. It's about slowing the mind down and keeping the spirit open.

We are what we practice, so if all you do is rush through your days, then your life is going to be a mess like that. We have to carve out time out of our days for pure, absolute nothingness. That is the highest form of productivity that there is. Stillness is what anchors us to our own intuition. There will always be that cacophony of voices around attempting to tell us who we should be, what we should be, and why we should be those things. When practicing stillness, you learn that the wisest voice that you can and should listen to is your own. Silencing all of those outside voices makes it easy for you to tap into your intuition and listen to what is true to you.

It improves your listening. Most people listen to provide responses, not to understand the person with whom they are engaged in conversation. In stillness, you learn that it is more important to hear what people are saying, instead of just wanting to talk all the time; in turn, you respond more empathetically and effectively, which helps you build richer and more rewarding relationships.

It helps you find clarity around situations that you find troubling. When your heart is troubled, the natural thing to want to do is try to find the solution, which often results in weeks of sleepless nights and endless anxiety. Stillness invites you to step back, to see the situation from a distance, instead of in the middle. There is clarity in distance. We will not always be able to change the situation that we are in, but there is always a solution, something that can help us move forward, despite all that is happening.

You are here. You have a story, and it is a part of a much greater story that is unfolding right now. You don't always have to have it all figured out. You don't always have to have all the answers. Keep yourself grounded in the truth that there is a higher power at work in your world. A power that will get you to where you are meant to be.

Bringing Stillness Into Everyday Moments

All it takes to incorporate stillness is a few moments throughout the day. It doesn't have to be complicated. Some of the ways through which you can incorporate it into your day include:

Finding stillness through every breath you take. There is power in breath. It's not just something that we do to keep ourselves alive, but something that we can use to reconnect with our higher selves; the ones that know better, make conscious decisions, and work towards being better every day.

Here is a simple breathing exercise you can follow to help you find your place as you learn to find your place within the practice.

- **Find a peaceful position to sit**. Make sure that your body is free of tension. Inhale deeply through the nose. Hold the inhale for at least five seconds, and then exhale, each one coming at a slow, steady pace. Continue with this rhythm until this breathing exercise feels natural and unforced. You don't have to think about anything as you do this.

- **Practice it as the moment requires**. Stillness is everywhere, regardless of what setting you are in. You can find it in your office in the middle of a busy day. Lock the door if you must and take a few minutes for yourself. This is a reminder to you that even amidst the hustle and bustle of your schedule, you can have calm and relaxing experiences everywhere you are.

- **Schedule it in your diary**. If it's something that you can't be spontaneous about, make that appointment with yourself. Make it a priority to honor this time that you are setting aside for yourself.

- **Start a journaling practice**. There is power in the written word. Nothing is quite as therapeutic as working through your thoughts and your emotions. You can be as unfiltered as you want to; there are no rules. It's just you, the pen between your fingers and the notebook right in front of you. The trick when journaling is to remain as self-aware as possible. Journalling is about creating something that is uniquely and beautifully yours, something that fits your personality. You should create something that you look forward to every day. So, don't worry about the small things such as barely legible handwriting, or spelling mistakes. Don't let those factors come in between you and what's inside your heart.

When journaling, it can be helpful to determine and analyze what is working and what isn't working when it comes to your journaling practice. Ask yourself what your journaling goals are. Do you want to be better at managing your stress and your anger? Look at those goals and evaluate what isn't working. If what you are currently doing right now isn't working, it's going to be difficult for you to turn journaling into an everyday habit, so take the time you need and experiment with what you want to find out which techniques work best for you. If the traditional pen and paper aren't working for you, you can switch to using your computer. If journaling isn't working in the morning, switch it up to the evenings or sometime in the afternoon when you have a moment to spare.

Lastly, it isn't always easy to come up with things to journal about. Words fail us all sometimes. That's why keeping a list of journal prompts can come in handy when you find yourself at a loss for words.

Journal Prompts for Moments of Reflection

• If I could list some of the best qualities there are about myself, which five things would be at the top of my list?

• Where would I like to see myself in the next coming year? What progress would I like to see myself making in the coming year?

• When was the last time I cried? Have I healed from that experience? If yes, what did it teach me, and if not, what steps can I take from here onward to try to be better for myself?

• What is the one thing that I've always been afraid to admit out loud? It could be a toxic relationship, a career change that I am afraid to make.

- What are some of my biggest aspirations, and what's holding me back from chasing those ambitions?
- Being where I am today, what pieces of advice would I give to my younger self?
- What three things would I like to change when it comes to my own personal development?
- What does the perfect morning look like for you? How does it feel when you wake up? When you look at the day ahead of you and all the activities lined up, what is it that you are looking forward to? Write about all that you would do during that perfect day. At noon, in the evening, and at nighttime?
- Reminisce about one of your favorite childhood memories. Why does this memory, in particular, bring you copious amounts of joy?
- What small, practical changes can you make to change your life for the better?
- Write about this moment. The details that surround it: sights, sounds, and smells included. What is it about it that makes it so... beautiful?

I guess you can say that I too am still learning how to breathe. I am still learning to not always turn my heart to the slightest sounds. I am learning to pace myself and not drown when there's chaos all around. Being alone truly is the biggest lesson that there is. You have all this time to grow as a person. Time to reflect on who you are as a person. Time to reflect on what you like and do not like about yourself. There is time to grow and flourish without a cacophony of unnecessary distractions.

We won't ever be able to create or give from places of emptiness, exhaustion, and uncertainty. For that to have you have to fill yourselves up, you have to let that generosity that you shower yourself with be the one that spills out into the world around you.

Chapter 5: Mind Your Tribe

Your soul people will find you, even if it's in moments that you least expect.

- **Human connection**. It's all about love. It's about sharing smiles and secret conversations, recipes, and secrets. It's about bringing Tupperware and Tupperware of food to friends in times of need. It's offering a hug to the one who is crying, it's rejoicing too when they have victories to share.

- **Sisterhood. Brotherhood**. Deep-rooted friendships can help us find support on this journey that we are on. When it comes from an authentic place of real love, joy, and authenticity, it gives our lives a depth that we could have never imagined. A richness that propels us forward and whispers to us that: together, we are better.

- **Connection matters**. Having loose ties and relationships with people other than ourselves can help conjure up more positive emotions and protect us from stress's negative effects on our lives. For example, getting a hug from a friend in a time of distress helps the brain produce feel-good hormones that can help you communicate feelings of gratefulness, empathy, and love. Feeling loved and accepted influences how we feel daily. Hugs, handholding, and words of affirmation, are all just as important as eating healthily, drinking enough water, and getting enough movement.

But just as much as we should push ourselves to get closer to people, it's just as important to be mindful of the quality of people that we are bringing in or allowing into our lives. Our connections can shape who we become biologically, which can be both good and bad. You are the sum of the people you surround yourself with because the people around us influence our views and opinions. The most noticeable ways that our people affect us are through their views, beliefs, habits, and behaviors. Even if you already have opinions of yours, hanging out with people with different views can alter the shape of our own beliefs, which isn't a negative thing, per se, but if they force us to go against our values, it might not be all that good for you.

They can either push you forward or stunt your growth. Those we spend our time with can either motivate or discourage us from chasing our dreams. Imagine having a friend who doesn't take themselves or their aspirations seriously, they are less likely to take your dreams seriously as well. Every time you talk about conquering the world of your fears, you'll be met with mockery; reactions that might make you feel as if your dreams are unattainable.

You'll either be filled with negative or positive emotions. Joy, love, excitement, and positivity are contagious, but so are hatred, negativity, pessimism, and a lack of gratitude. If you are surrounded by people who never seem to stop complaining, it's going to take a real toll on your mental health, you'll feel exhausted for no reason, you'll find yourself feeling bitter, and more so, you may even start complaining as well just to fit in.

Your joy and your happiness will be affected. The people you are surrounded by can have an impact on how satisfied you truly feel with your life. If the people you hang out with make you feel as if you are insignificant or less than others, it's going to impact the way that you view yourself, you might find yourself wanting to change everything about yourself, or doing things that you don't want to do to fit in a crowd that doesn't matter all that much. Research shows that the quality of our friendships has a significant effect on our levels of satisfaction in life.

"I hear you. I see you, and I choose to welcome you as you are."

"All of you are welcome here. The whole parts, the messy ones, and the parts that are not all that easy to understand as well." When we are in the presence of people who welcome inclusivity, people who aren't afraid of realness, it allows us to break the cycle of thinking that we need to change ourselves to be accepted.

There are people who are for us and ones who aren't. All of our work here on earth is in service of a deep connection, whether it's bringing ourselves together with people through music, art, or intimate conversations.

Finding Your Tribe

- **Choosing who your friends are is incredibly important.** At the end of the day, you want to find yourself with people who will stick around not only during the good times but through the bad times as well. You want people who are magic bringers, light chasers, and people whose heartbeats are in sync with yours.

- **Find friends who are honest.** You need people who tell you what you need to hear and not just what you want to hear. You need friends who are capable of saying the tough things as much as they are capable of showering you with compliments and words that speak lightly. Honest friends are the ones who keep from walking away when the doubt starts kicking in.

- **Find the ones who give just as much as they take.** Reciprocation is important in friendships and relationships. They're about compromise. Choose friends who are willing to make time for you as much as you make time for them. One-sided friendships often lead to a whole lot of bottled-up anger and resentment. It's all about balance because balance is healthy.

- **Find people who understand why your values are important to you.** I have come to learn a lot about respect. Respect teaches us that regardless of who we are or where we come from, we all matter. It's okay to have friends whose values are different from our own. The way they see things is just as important as the way we see things. Our values are what keep us anchored to who we are.

- **Find friends who are your partners on purpose.** Fill your circle with people who are able to hold down intellectual and casual conversations. I want to have friends with whom I can have conversations about finances, career, and personal growth as well as the silly conversations about why I didn't like last night's episode of gray's anatomy, or why vanilla lattes are a thousand times better than the pumpkin spice ones. So, what do the conversations with your current circle feel and look like? Sit on that for a while and when you are ready to give yourself the answer, ask yourself if their company is supporting the growth mindset that you are cultivating.

• **Find friends who are doing better than you**. As people, we rarely want to find ourselves around people who are doing better than us, which is understandable because no one really wants to feel like they're behind or not doing enough. It's okay to step outside of our comfort zones every now and again, sometimes to figure out what it is that we want and do not want. We need to find ourselves in foreign territory. Perspective is everything when you are still figuring things out.

You and I both know our weaknesses, so find the people who can compliment you in those areas. The right friends can help you dig into your raw and untapped potential. Perhaps you are a friend that's a gifted wordsmith, so why not use that skill and help that friend in need polish their resume or update their LinkedIn portfolio? Relationships and friendships are about winning together, so in return, they can help you win at something by using their strengths to help you.

Find the ones with an insatiable hunger for knowledge. The greatest conversations that I've had have been with people who are avid readers. I love literature. From classical and contemporary fiction to self-help. I love the idea that some gifted writer created an entire book using words strung together as sentences to keep my mind entertained and alive; stories that create a gallery of my mind—a place where I can't return to remind myself of the healing powers of art—literature is the greatest reminder there is that we will figure it out, and even if we don't, we'll make it out okay to the other side.

When we were a lot younger, we believed that it was much better to be part of the popular. In some ways, we do that as adults as well. We think that being part of the elite will make our lives a lot easier (which is true to a certain extent). You shouldn't have to sacrifice much to keep the friends you have. You shouldn't have to sacrifice your intelligence, your values, and your sense of dignity in the name of friendship.

If the crowd is what you choose to follow, you eventually are going to end up losing yourself. But when you choose to lose the crowd and follow your soul instead, you'll find that the soul tribe eventually does appear; that existing in temporary solitude is okay if the people aren't for you.

Letting Go of Relationships Don't Serve You

Here are some words of advice for you. Stop trying to take people to places that they don't deserve to go with you. It's okay to leave them where they are and forge ahead with your life because sometimes, to keep yourself held together, you have to allow yourself to leave, even if it breaks you just a little. Peace is sometimes about doing things that aren't easy.

They are not good for you if:

- You dread interactions with them. You spend hours or days before feeling anxious and worried sick.
- You replay conversations that you have with them over and over and over again in your head because you worry that you might not have said the right thing or that what you said might make them upset with you or something like that.
- You can't be yourself when you are around them.
- You feel the need to de-stress after interactions with them, usually through alcohol, excessive eating, or smoking.
- You complain to others about them.

It's easier to want to stick with a friendship because it's a lot easier than sticking with it and not dealing with the issues head-on. But in doing that, you don't realize that you are actually robbing yourself of valuable energy and time that can be better utilized elsewhere. You don't have to hate yourself for cutting yourself off from relationships that lead to you hating yourself.

Stop putting your worth in your friendships. You are not your friend. Stop buying into the idea that the more friends you have, the happier you'll be. A good friend is far more valuable than a million if they are the right one.

You don't have to explain yourself to them. I've talked myself out of doing things more times than I have actually talked myself into doing things because I don't always want to have those tough conversations. What would I say in those moments? What would they even think of me? The great thing, however, is that we all have the power of choice, so you can be selective with what you choose or choose not to say. You'll struggle in the beginning, but as you get yourself used to the idea, you'll find that it's not as difficult as it seems.

Your gut knows best. Are you in touch with your intuition—those little tingles in your stomach that tell you that something might be a little off? That feeling resides there for a reason, and we have an obligation to work on that relationship with it because it's our guiding light—divine intervention—if you prefer referring to it in that way. Regardless of how subtle it is, if it gives you an indication that it's time for you to go, acknowledge its truth and go with it.

Try not to shift the blame. When things aren't going well, in life, friendship or otherwise, it's natural to want to cast the blame on someone else. They're the ones who brought so and so into your life, so if it weren't for them, you wouldn't be in the predicament that you are in. Doing this only feeds into our own inner self-sabotage and makes it more difficult for us to move on. People are who they show us to be. If that is something that we are not willing to accept, we'll only continue blaming ourselves for their actions. That hardly seems fair, don't you think?

Don't remain bitter for too long. The last thing you want to do is rob yourself of an opportunity to experience joy past that friendship. Harboring bitterness is the equivalent of drinking acid and expecting the other person to sustain the injuries, create that distance that you need and when your heart does heal, forgive them, free yourself from any guilt, and move on. You deserve that much, don't you think?

Accept that sometimes the apology you are waiting for might never come because they might think that there is nothing wrong that they did, so why apologize? The quicker it is that you accept that, the easier it will be for you to move on with your life.

You can allow yourself to grieve the ending of the friendship. I sometimes refer to my friendships (the good and the bad ones) as a portfolio of my life. There are precious memories embedded in the moments of these relationships. You allowed yourself to be vulnerable, to be happy, and excited about these people. You invested time and energy within these interactions, so it's understandable why nostalgia might creep in, or why you might have a bit of a tough time letting go. Allow yourself to grieve those cherished memories that you made. The weight of that sadness does lighten after a while.

Not all toxic people have cruel intentions. Some of them do love us, and dearly so. But just because that is the case, it still doesn't mean that they are good for us. Life is already hard as it is; why make it any harder by putting yourself in the presence of people who are constantly trying to bring you down?

Not everyone who comes into your life is meant to stay there, so when the time's right, I can only hope that you are brave enough to let go.

Chapter 6: Romancing Yourself

If I had a dollar for every time someone asked me: "Do you love yourself?" I'd be filthy rich. The obvious answer to give is yes, and for good reason. The last thing that anybody wants to admit is that they don't really love themselves.

Pleasure matters in life. It matters because it's what makes the mundane, or not-so-pleasant moments and turns them into pockets of joy and pleasure. Pleasure—it's singing and dancing off-beat as your favorite song blares through the speaker. It's letting your favorite candle burn as you read your comfort book. It's making space for the things that matter to you, things that you enjoy amidst all the things that you "have to" do.

Self-love, however, is more than just pampering yourself with gifts and dining out at fancy restaurants. It's getting to know yourself at a deeper level. Doing things that you are not all that comfortable with. It's being patient about the fact that the growth that you are looking for is not going to magically happen overnight. It's remembering to constantly remind yourself that change doesn't come easily; that you have to be willing to brave it through the scariest bits.

Learning to love yourself is learning that you don't have to hold yourself prisoner to any past mistakes that you made when you didn't know any better. Self-love is about learning to be aware of your emotions so that you don't subject yourself to endless servings of judgment and self-criticism.

Self-love is about forgiveness. It enables you to extend much-needed grace so that you can move forward with yourself. So that you can understand the reasons behind the things that you do.

It teaches you acceptance and that, I believe, is the cornerstone of all great progress. The home of all unconditional love. Acceptance is about realizing that one bad day or bad a week does not mean that your entire life is doomed. It's about knowing that you can have days where you are both upset and not feeling your best self, but deciding that you'll try again tomorrow, and again on the days to come because embracing the fullness of life means welcoming both the sadness and joy, all alike.

Whether you are in a relationship or still exploring your own sexuality, you deserve to have a strong, healthy, and intimate relationship with yourself. That is how you build and strengthen your self-esteem. How you learn to stand up for yourself even when you are the only one traveling along that path that you are on. You do it so that you don't grow resentful in your relationships so that you have more compassion, and a healthier perspective, and that you learn to make decisions that YOU can benefit from; choices that have your best interests in mind.

Some might say that self-love is a little conceited or selfish, but that is far from the truth. Loving ourselves well equips us with that dash of magic that enables us to love those around us in the ways that they too, deserve to be loved.

Learning to Love Yourself

The best parts of life are in those seemingly unnoticeable moments in life when you realize that getting to know yourself on an intimate and intimate level is something that you never want to stop doing.

- **Nourish yourself.** That is the best place to start, in my opinion. If you are totally new to this whole concept of self-love, the best place where you can start is with your body, because the body is what takes us from place to place. What keeps us alive and sustains us in some ways in which you can show your body the love that it deserves:
- **Movement.** It doesn't have to be those complex movements that you see all these YouTube and Instagram models doing to be considered worthy enough. You don't have to go to the gym five times a week to enjoy all the full benefits of movement. Moderate activities such as walking, swimming, and yoga will serve as much justice as a full-body workout in the gym. Other sneaky ways that you can get yourself a good workout without even realizing, are by parking further away from entrances when you go to the shopping center, cleaning, and even cooking!
- **Fuel the right way.** The food that we eat has such a great impact on how we feel, so you want to make sure that you are eating foods that are leaving you energized and giving your body all the nutrients that it needs. In saying this, I am not saying that you should be cutting out all of your favorite foods from your diet. Moderation is key when developing a healthy lifestyle. It's okay if on some days you feel like having the fruit salad, and others feel like having the slice of chocolate cake. Depriving ourselves does more harm than good, so learn to savor the delicacies that you love to eat so that you can actually enjoy them!
- **Take yourself on a date!** Solo dating is all about getting to know yourself better. It's about spending quality time with yourself so that you can figure out what it is that you enjoy doing, and also to help you enjoy the moments that you spend in the company of those you care for. By

doing something that you wouldn't normally do, you are making a bold declaration of how it is you know you deserve to be loved. So, what exactly do you do when you woo yourself? Anything that leaves you buzzing or evokes that tingly feeling that comes from falling in love.

○ Put on a comfy outfit and go on a nature walk. You can even forage for some pretty flowers or greenery to decorate your house with.

○ Visit a local museum or art gallery.

○ Sign up to be a volunteer at an orphanage or a shelter that serves a cause that you are passionate about. This might not sound like it's something that you'd typically do for a date but believe me when I say this—you are going to feel so much better.

○ Grab a book and go and sit in your local cafe to read (perfect place and time to exhibit serious main character energy).

○ Go all out and cook yourself an extravagant three-course meal.

○ If you feel like splurging a little, you can book yourself in a fancy hotel

○ and go and watch a live music show or a concert.

○ If you are a daredevil enough, go skydiving or bungee jumping. The list is really endless. If it's something that you would say yes to doing with a partner, go ahead and do it all by yourself.

● **Be kinder to yourself.** This seems like an easy enough thing to matter, but when we're being honest with each other, it's actually one of the most difficult things there is to master because of this certain level of perfectionism that society expects us to uphold. You don't have to be the super mom who sometimes sends her kids to school with pre-packaged dinners or sometimes makes freezer dinners for her family because she's had a long day at work and can't seem to muster up the energy to start peeling and chopping vegetables. You don't have to have the body of a full-time fitness trainer to be worthy of love. You are a human. Not some man-made robot that should be expected to produce perfect results all the time. Be kind to yourself; this is my permission slip to you.

○ Give yourself the recognition you deserve. Did you just beat a personal best in an early morning run? Go ahead and give yourself a high five. Did you just get a promotion at work? Go ahead and write that letter to yourself detailing how proud it is that you really are of yourself. You don't have to wait for someone else to tell you what a fine job it is that you've done.

○ Advocate for yourself. Your inner advocate is the tiny voice that steps in when the inner critic wants to take in. it's the voice that jumps in and presents an argument on your behalf.

○ Forgive yourself. Nobody goes through life without a couple of misses. Maybe there's something that you did that you are not entirely proud of. Perhaps you struggled to stand up for yourself and let someone walk all over you. Maybe a great opportunity slipped from your fingers because you let your fear get the best of you. You don't have to continue blaming yourself for the things that you did when you didn't know better. Make a promise to yourself that you are going to do better and move on from there.

○ Don't stop reminding yourself of all the other good qualities that you possess. You may be terrible at numbers, but hey, you are a gifted wordsmith or pretty artistic. you may sometimes be over dramatic but, don't forget about that sense of humor that is capable of bringing life to rooms and any situation. For every flaw that you are tempted to point out, there are always three more things that outweigh it.

● **Say no more often**. You are not obligated to dish out a lengthy explanation at any given time when you choose to say no to something.

○ No, I don't feel comfortable doing that.

○ No, I do not feel like attending that gathering.

○ No, this is something I'd rather not do because it does not align with my values.

○ No, this does make me feel happy.

Saying no is empowering. It gives you the freedom to own your time and your space. So, remember that you do not have to say yes to anything that you feel is an invasion of your space. You shouldn't strive to accommodate people if it compromises your woman's happiness.

● **Be compassionate**. If you were your friend, sister, brother, or your child, what things would you say to them to make them feel a little better? What kind of treatment would you give them, and what reassurance would you give to reassure them that they are loved? Now take those answers, translate them into a love language of your own, and do those things for yourself.

The secret to a revolutionary kind of self-love is making your opinion about yourself the center of your world; it's about caring less about what other people think about you and focusing more on what you think about yourself. I don't always like myself when I focus my gaze on the reflection in the mirror, sometimes I need that extra push, through a verse a poem, a song—any form or reassurance, if that is what you are feeling today, here are some reminders to keep you going:

• It's okay if I am struggling to love myself today. Regardless of those feelings, I will be as kind to myself as I can.

• I am lucky that I get to be me. There are multiple reminders of life all around me that serve as my daily reminders of how blessed I am.

• Joy is something that I deserve to experience on a daily basis. So, I am going to strive to work intentionally toward it every day.

• Releasing stress is relatively easy when I remind myself to relax and breathe. And right now, this is what I am choosing to do.

• I am a good person. And because of that, goodness continually chooses to chase after and find me.

• Today, I am choosing to harness the power of acceptance. I am embracing all that I am and all that I am feeling at this current moment. Even when it's hard, I know that I will make it out stronger on the other side.

• I choose to be patient with myself and with the progress that I am making, when I intentionally choose the pace for myself that best suits my life. That is how I take my power back.

Take the scenic route in your life. Say "I love you" to yourself and say it often. Recite poems in your head that only you understand the meaning of. Eat pastries and desserts whose names you struggle to pronounce. Chase sunrises and sunsets, and forage for joy in the most unlikely of places. Sing and make music from the holiest place within your belly. These precious moments are all the necessary salt of life. Chase after them unapologetically. Your life is the story, and you—the main character, so treat yourself like the royalty that you are.

Chapter 7: Trim, Trim, Trim

We have all experienced those days. You sleep past the sound of your alarm or maybe you snoozed one too many times, and just as you are about to leave, spill coffee all over the outfit that you spent the entire evening ironing. And just as you thought things couldn't get any worse, you find traffic on the way to work. You arrive at the office thinking that your luck for the day might change—you sit down at your desk committed to remaining in your center because surely you are just being tested. Cue the phone call because you check your planner and it dawns on you that you have got a full day of meetings lined up for the day, that's not even the worst of it because you've been procrastinating on a couple of projects, all of which are due in the next two days how did you get here? How could you let them get so out of hand?

So, what do you do when everything on your To-Do list seems important? What do you do to make up for all that time that you seemingly lost? Or what do you do when you just can't seem to find that sweet spot where you feel as if you have control over your life?

I can't tell you what balance is because it's a combination of multiple things. It might mean making time for your fitness, your dating life, your friends, or blissful relaxation. I can't say that I'm a pro when it comes to.

Managing my time or prioritizing tasks so that I am more efficient and productive throughout the day. Some days I spend lounging on the couch, binge-watching series, even when I do realize that my time could be better used elsewhere.

- **Time is invaluable**. We all have equal access to it, but why does it seem that some people have more of it than others? It's simple. Time management. The better you are at planning ahead, the less you'll rush. Things that used to overwhelm you will feel effortless.
- **Schedule your time**. You can use a calendar, a bullet journal, or a piece of paper. Figure out what tasks you need to do throughout the week. These can include work deadlines, errands that you need to run,

meetings that you need to attend, and any other personal commitments that you need to attend throughout the week. Split the activities on the days of the week. When doing this, be sure to not over-allocate too many tasks in one day. The goal is to get as much done as you can without overwhelming or overworking yourself to the bone.

- **Determine the urgency of the task.** Not everything that is important is urgent. Urgent means that it requires immediate attention. Important tasks are the ones that contribute to the long-term goals that are in service of your mission or your goals.

- **Put similar tasks together.** To preserve your energy, you can block out time on your calendar to do certain things like respond to emails, make follow-up calls, or respond to messages. Avoid responding to your messages or your emails as they come in. This tends to divert your attention from the task that you are busy with at the moment, making it an even longer one to complete.

- **Make time limits for yourself.** The perfectionist in you says that you cannot stop working on the task at hand until you've nailed it down to a T. This is self-sabotage at best because it prevents you from doing tasks that you were planning on completing. You might even start to feel as if you are making no progress at all. Time management is about creating a steady workflow for yourself. So having stints in between tasks reduces the mental strain that you put on yourself and can help you keep your motivation consistent. (i.e., If you are working on creative projects, like designing or writing, schedule time for first drafts, revisions, and final deliverables),

- **Optimize your energy levels.** When are you most productive throughout the day? It's important to keep a tab on your body's energy fluctuations throughout the day. So, are you more productive in the earlier times of the day, or are you most productive in the afternoon? So, make the most of that and use that time to complete your most challenging tasks. This will allow you to complete and deliver high-quality work in less time.

Ways You Can Boost Your Energy Levels

Don't skimp on those zzz's. So many people cut corners on their sleep to meet deadlines, to get on more study time, and the side effects of that often result in grumpiness and feeling tired the next day—so essentially cutting down on your sleep to get more done, ends up doing more harm than good. If you are having trouble sleeping, try implementing some of these techniques:

- **Have a consistent bedtime.** If your sleep schedule is all over the place, you'll benefit by having a consistent bedtime. Allow your body to get into the rhythm of waking up and going to bed at the same time each day.

- **Less light.** Make adjustments to the lighting in your room to allow you to sleep better. Use candles, fairy lights, or night lights. Harsh, bright lighting often disturbs our bodies' sleep cycles, creating a more atmospheric environment for yourself, and putting your body in that relaxed state that can help you ease into that relaxed state of quality sleep.

- **Read or listen to an audiobook,** or a podcast. Reading is a great way to take your mind away from the chaos around you. It helps you release that build-up of stress that made its way into your body throughout the day and makes it easier for you to fall asleep. If reading doesn't tickle your fancy, audiobooks or podcasts, work just as big a wonder as a traditional book.

- **Unplug yourself.** It's relaxing to spend those last few hours of your evening browsing through your Instagram or Facebook or to send off one final email for the day. That blue light that is emitted from the screen of your cellphone blocks the production of melatonin, which makes you sleepy. Ideally, you should be putting your devices to rest an hour before you go to bed.

- **Watch your caffeine throughout the day.** If you are sensitive to caffeine, it's best to watch how much caffeine you are ingesting mid-afternoon.

- **Be mindful of how much and what you are eating before your bedtime**. Avoid eating heavy meals three hours before your bedtime. This will give your body enough time to digest the food. If you are looking to have a light snack, I would recommend foods such as yogurt, berries, almonds/ nuts, or bananas.

- **Take advantage of the productivity tools that there are**. A productivity tool is an application that helps you optimize your tasks. Some examples include Calendly, which helps you schedule the tasks that you need to do and keep track of meetings and other commitments that you need to attend to. Trello—it's a project management tool that helps organize your workflow by creating detailed lists of the tasks that you need to do.

- **Delegate your tasks effectively**. You do not have to do everything by yourself. If there is someone you know who can do the task at hand just as efficiently as you can, ask them to do it while you focus on other things.

- **Avoid multitasking**. When you multitask, it may look and feel as though you are doing more with your time, but that is not the case. Doing too many things at one time causes you to lose focus, which leads to you making bigger mistakes, which takes you back to square one, giving you more work than you had initially bargained for.

- **Rest**. It's just as productive as completing another task. Resting is what helps you improve your performance. Not taking breaks will only result in feelings of restlessness, which makes it take longer to finish your tasks. Give yourself at least 20 minutes where you stretch your legs and listen to your body and how it's communicating with you. If it tells you that it's time to stop. Stop. It's what allows you to do all that you are doing right now. To honor and respect it, give it what it needs at that moment.

- **Minimize the distractions around you as you get your work done**. It's easier to keep your focus when there are not a bunch of things around you demanding your attention. Distractions can be both physical and digital. The digital ones include your cell phone and social media, and the physical ones include clutter or working in an overcrowded space. So, some of the things that you can do to help you endure that you'll keep your attention span for as long as possible are:

○ Making your workspace less cluttered. Keep only things that are functional and practical.

○ Muting our push notifications.

○ Using noise-canceling headphones.

Being organized is your way of bringing more joy back into your life. It's how you reclaim your freedom and joy. Life really is a lot less complicated when we decide to take responsibility when we choose when we decide that the choice lies with us. We are the ones who have the power of choice. Blindly following or jumping on the bandwagon of the status quo without knowing why that thing is important to us only sets us back and stalls our progress.

Instead of working against your wiring, why not work with it, instead? March to the beat of your own drum. It's in and of itself a lovely melody, even if it's slightly offbeat.

Chapter 8: Taking Full Accountability

I love it when I am brave enough to admit that sometimes I am the cause of my own problems. This realization brings me to another big realization, that I am the solution to the problems that I sometimes create for myself. Progress and humility go hand in hand. You cannot move forward if you are continuously playing the blame game. You have to step up and admit that sometimes you are a toxic person in your own life.

What is Personal accountability and why is it such an important aspect when creating an intentional life? Personal accountability is following through on everything that you say you will do for yourself. It's managing the expectations that you have of yourself, being proactive, thinking strategically, and aiming toward more consistently.

Here Are a Few Things to Remember About Accountability:

It's hard because we associate it with perfectionism, and at the root of all perfectionism, is judgment and shame. Perhaps you grew up in a household where your parents constantly told you that you were not doing enough, that number two wasn't good enough, and that you always had to strive to get to that first place. Accountability isn't about perfection, perfection tells you that you are not allowed to make mistakes, it tells you that you are not acceptable as you are, that your worth is something that needs to be earned; either in the form of status or unrealistic expectations that you impose upon yourself. To me accountability is a lot like that loving parent who waits on their doorstep with arms wide open and welcomes back their prodigal child back home, regardless of what you've done, it tells you that you have worth here; it invites us to hold space for curiosity, to reflect on that situation that was and ask yourself in the future, what is it that I can do differently next time?

It requires you to be a master at self-forgiveness. As your capacity to forgive yourself expands, your outlook to look forward to the future will grow as well. Self-forgiveness serves that unhealthy bond that we have with perfectionism. Granting ourselves that permission to not be perfect, but simply human, rebuilds that road toward self-trust and gives us permission to do things. I haven't always been in this place where I can find peace within myself. Somehow, I thought that beating myself up for days on end about something I did would change what happened—it didn't work then, and it still doesn't work now. So, if you needed a reminder today, I hope you realize that it is okay to forgive yourself. You are allowed to forgive yourself for all those times when you didn't know better because you can, at any given time, turn into the best you that you've ever been. You didn't know then what you know now, and mistakes are how you get your second chances. Here are a few tips on how you can practice some self-forgiveness.

- **Process your emotions**. Our emotional triggers are difficult to face. I've given myself the permission that you need to gradually welcome them, meet them, and familiarize yourself with them so that you can eventually move forward.

- **Unburden yourself by voicing that mistake out loud**. Putting a name to that scenario in mind will help you learn from it so that you don't repeat that same mistake sometime again in the future.

- **Engage in those conversations with your inner critic**. Communicating with that part of you that makes you so hard on yourself can help you develop an attitude of self-compassion towards yourself. Use a journal or a diary to highlight those patterns of thinking that make it particularly difficult for you to forgive yourself.

- **You can work through it with a professional**. There is no shame in seeking help from a professional who can help you come up with better and healthier strategies to cope. Even the strongest people need a helping hand every now and again—you included.

Something else I'd like you to remember is that accountability is not something that you can pass on to someone else. There is nothing wrong with having a role model or a mentor, but those people are not responsible for the decisions that you make. They're there to give you advice, and it's up to you to decide how you apply their teachings in your life. Sure, you'll feel a lot better telling yourself: I got this wrong because you told me to do it this way. Is it helping you in any way or form to become better?

It becomes a lot easier to be patient with yourself when you are aware of your self-sabotaging behaviors and habits. It also makes it easier for you to set goals for yourself to work towards. Acknowledging your growth points and clarifying where it is that you want to spend more of your time reminds you to keep your focus when drifting astray.

Chapter 9: A map To Joy-Finding

My wish for you: A joy that glitters despite all circumstances...

Dear Joy,

Come into my life uninvited and as you wish. I want you to know that your presence is something that should feel like no stranger to me. I want to know you well. I want you to be my best friend. I want to take you places with me. And if I ever do find myself in a place where I feel empty and drained of all life, I want to know without certainty that I can always reach a hand out to you because there are about a million little ways in which our presence is capable of reviving a tired soul.

I am a glutton for joy. There is no passion within me that burns as fiercely as the one that depicts my love for joy. And I do believe without a doubt that joy leaves pieces of itself within us so that even in our moments of weakness, we know that there is a place of love within us that we can always return to when we need it the most.

Joy is something that all of us want in life, but it's hard because we are so afraid that it can be taken away from us so easily as well. There is this mentality that it is fleeting and is going to be taken away from us at any moment from now so why bother trying, why bother when you might only just experience it for a couple of seconds and have it snatched away from you in seconds like it never mattered at all. It is courageous for someone to decide that they are going to experience joy just because they can.

Your joy is attached to material possessions, or it is dependent upon the acceptance of others. Joy in its purest is manufactured in the heart. It will never be a constant for you if your experience of it is dependent on what does and doesn't happen. Joy doesn't have a reason. You are allowed to feel it just because... Just because you love how the sun lights up your room in the afternoons. Just because you are happy to be here today. Breathing, putting one foot in front of another. Your joy can be as big or as small as you want it to be.

You compare yourself too much to other people. People share what they want you to see. They may look like they are happy on the outside, but are they really? Just because they look one hundred times happier than you, it does not mean they are. Stop trying to "out joy" other people. Your joy is not their joy, and theirs is not yours. Experience yours in the unique way that it shows up.

Your Habits of Joy

Joy is something that you continuously work towards. Sometimes I like to think to myself that it kind of falls unexpectedly into your hands unexpectedly and chooses to stay there. But it doesn't work like that. It doesn't choose us based on who we are. We choose it ourselves because we know that it is for all of us.

Stop waiting for someday. I am going to feel more joyful when I finally get my position. I am going to feel more joyful when I finally graduate. I know joy will come much easier when I eventually buy that house or that car... So, for now, I will pretend that I am okay and hope the worst doesn't happen... Joy doesn't work like that. You can still obtain all of those things but not feel any happier. Chances are your moment to be happy has already come right past you, but you let it slip by because you were too busy waiting for someday to notice it. Don't be that person.

Appreciate the small things. Oh, how we take those things for granted. We overlook these things that are capable of making our lives so, so beautiful. We let them slip right past us and consider ourselves the forgotten souls, but joy isn't selfish. She caters to everyone.

If you are in search of inspiration, enjoy my list to you of the tiny, magnificent things that make life absolutely blissful:

- Laying underneath the stars at night, stargazing, and philosophizing about life.
- Laughing until you cry or randomly fart.
- Having breakfast in bed or enjoying a full morning of doing pure nothingness in bed.
- Tasting something magnificent for the first time.
- Being the first person in line at a coffee shop in town on a busy morning.
- The smell of freshly mown grass wafting in your window.
- Pressing your fingers in bubble wrap.

- Dropping something accidentally but finding it unscathed and untouched.
- Slipping into a pair of pants that fit as perfectly as a glove.
- Giving someone who's hard to please good love.
- Seeing a cute guy or a girl.
- Being able to pursue creative endeavors
- That lightbulb moment when you realize that all your work for the day is complete, and you can spend the rest of the day doing anything you want.
- Hopping into a bed that has been made with freshly ironed sheets.
- Holding something in your hands that you've wanted for a long time.
- Seeing clouds that look like the face of someone or something that you recognize.

These things that I have listed here for you are just some of the many places where you can start. To maximize the power and effects that these little things have in your life, you should definitely try weaving them into your routine or moments in your everyday life. The more of them you have around, the more pleasant your life will be.

Also, don't limit yourself to the ones that we've mentioned above. Create your own list. The things that you add to that list don't have to make sense to me or anyone else if it is something that adds color to the patches of gray in your life. Keep them there.

You don't have to buy your way to joy. Life has it in abundance and she is willing to offer it to us if we are.

Conclusion

I set out to write this book because I wanted to leave people with something that would make them feel good about themselves. Having spent years getting in the way of my own peace, I spent a lot of time wondering what it would look and feel like to be content with where and who I am. Stop waiting on other people to tell me that this is what you should do. To stop waiting for validation. To let go of the mentality that I had to pinpoint my joy to a specific reason. To be alive, full of life, love, and vitality, and to hug myself despite what was and wasn't happening around me.

You are good enough. You are worthy enough. You are perfect, wonderful just as you are, right where you are. You don't have to guilt yourself into change. All I know is that forcing yourself to be some kind of different rarely ever works. All changes that you want to take place must come from a place of love within you. I hope that this book is something that you can continuously return to when the noise of the world gets too loud, or when you think that you aren't doing enough, or moving fast enough to achieve all of your goals. I hope that this book can be your sanctuary, your place of ease and love and rest.

A Few Final Heartful Reminders to Rest Your Heart Upon

Be soft with yourself today, tomorrow, and forevermore. That is my one wish for you today. You deserve a full, uninterrupted evening of rest. You deserve all the reminders, words of encouragement, and unconditional love that there is there for you.

Life is not a script. There's always time to learn, to find yourself, to explore, and see new sides of the world that you never knew existed. Take your sweet time and shape your life and while you are at it, don't forget to stop and enjoy the views that you encounter along the way.

I want you to remember too that doing your best on a daily basis will look different on a daily basis. Sometimes rest will be the best that you can do, and that to me is pretty good enough.

You are not a failure if things don't go the way you want them to.

It's easier to leave the chair beside you unoccupied, rather than opening it up for anyone who comes along. Don't undervalue the company you keep. If you haven't found your people yet, don't be disheartened. Someday, you'll cross paths with the ones who make you feel incredibly alive and cared for.

You are allowed to wake up one day and decide that you want to change and want to change. That you want to change the way in which you do things. You don't have to stay a certain way because you are afraid that people will judge you or won't accept this version of you that they are not familiar with.

Someone asked me a while ago what my biggest fear was. I sat on the question for a while because I wasn't sure how to respond. And then it hit me, coming to the end of my life and realizing that I let my life slip right past my fingers. For as long as I am here, I want to grip the entirety of my life with both of my hands. So, when you look in stillness at the canvas of your life, I hope you realize that the big good stuff in life exists in these moments right now.

May you be well, friend. May you be healthy, happy, and content.

Take care!

Glossary

Accountability: The act of taking responsibility for something.

Balanced lifestyle: Taking into consideration all aspects of your life (relationships, work, fitness, and health) and ensuring that they help you lead a life that you can keep up with.

Compassion: showing your concern when others aren't in good fortune.

Emotional Regulation: Your ability to manage your emotions well in situations of adversity

Emotional Triggers: Factors in your life that cause you severe distress. They are often characterized by crying uncontrollably, panicking, or uncontrollable anxiety.

Empathy: being able to identify with the thoughts and struggles of another.

Habits: Behaviors that you practice consistently.

Health: The overall physical, emotional, and mental state of an individual.

Priorities: Things in one's life that are more important than others

Self-Care: Taking your mental, emotional, and physical well-being into your hands by engaging in behaviors that increase your capacity to experience joy and satisfaction in life.

Self-Compassion: Being kind and understanding towards ourselves when we struggle.

Self-Help: Using the resources that are available to you to better yourself or overcome challenges that you encounter.

Wellness: Engaging in behaviors that serve to preserve your health.

References

Blone, V. (2022, January 17). *How to Make Time For Everything Without Getting Stressed*. Vishaka Blone. https://vishakablone.com/make-time-for-everything/

Davis, T. (n.d.). *Your Personal Values: What Are Values and How Do You Live Them?* The Berkeley Well-Being Institute. https://www.berkeleywellbeing.com/your-personal-values.html

Eatough, E. (2022, May 13). *How to Set Goals and Achieve Them: 10 Strategies for Success*. Www.betterup.com. https://www.betterup.com/blog/how-to-set-goals-and-achieve-them?hsLang=en

Express. (2016, October 6). *REVEALED: The Top 50 Things Most Likely To Make YOU Smile*. Express.co.uk. https://www.express.co.uk/life-style/life/718333/Top-50-things-make-you-smile

Green Drop. (n.d.). *Minimalism: Understanding Its Most Important Principles*. GoGreenDrop Blog. https://www.gogreendrop.com/blog/minimalism-understanding-its-most-important-principles/

Karr, A. (2017, December 15). *9 Simple Ways to Be Happy Every Day*. Canadian Living. https://www.canadianliving.com/health/mind-and-spirit/article/9-simple-ways-to-be-happy-every-day

LeMind, A., & B.A. (2021, December 6). *5 Reasons You Are Who You Hang Out With*. The Power of Misfits.

https://powerofmisfits.com/mind/you-are-who-you-hang-out-with/

PeopleHum. (2022, December 16). *Difference Between Urgent and Important Tasks*. Peoplehum. https://www.peoplehum.com/blog/the-divide-between-urgent-and-important-tasks

Popplestone, T. (2016, December 8). *30 Things You Can Do To Live More Simply*. Mindbodygreen. https://www.mindbodygreen.com/articles/ways-to-live-more-simply

Pure Heart Designs. (n.d.). *Healthy Living at Home: 7 Interior Design Tips*. Pure Haven Designs. Retrieved January 8, 2023, from https://www.purehavends.com/blog/healthy-living-at-home-7-interior-design-tips

Robbins, M. (2021, October 25). *The Importance of Self-Trust*. Mike-Robbins.com. https://mike-robbins.com/the-importance-of-self-trust/

Smith, S. (n.d.). *Why You Struggle with Accountability and How to Actually Change*. GrowthSource Coaching. https://www.growthsourcecoaching.com/why-you-struggle-with-accountability-and-how-to-actually-change.html

Steber, C. (2016, May 6). *11 Tips For Letting Go Of A Toxic Friendship, Even If It Seems Impossible*. Bustle; Bustle. https://www.bustle.com/articles/159131-11-tips-for-letting-go-of-a-toxic-friendship-even-if-it-seems-impossible

Treadgold, G. (n.d.). Page. Incafrica.com. https://incafrica.com/library/gordon-tredgold-7-truths-about-accountability-that-you-need-to-kno

Valley Schools. (2021, December 17). *The Importance of Human Connection*. Valley Schools. https://myvalleyschools.org/the-importance-of-human-connection/

Williams, J.-R. (2018, March 18). *Letting Go of Friends and How To Do it Without Hating Yourself.* Jessica Rose Williams. https://www.jessicarosewilliams.com/journal/letting-go-of-friends-and-how-to-do-it-without-hating-yourself

Your Life, Your Voice. (n.d.). *9 Steps to Taking Care of Yourself. Your Life Your Voice.* Retrieved January 8, 2023, from https://www.yourlifeyourvoice.org/Pages/tip-9-steps-to-taking-care-of-yourself.aspx